Waiting for Success

Johanne Mesidor-Dorsainvil

RN, BSN

Dedication

This book is dedicated to my husband Enel and my beautiful sister Diana. Thank you both for supporting me in continuation of my project. Despite obstacles, you two allowed me to dream that all is possible through God.

Waiting for Success

Johanne Mesidor-Dorsainvil RN, BSN

Copyright © 2018 Johanne Mesidor-Dorsainvil

Self-Published

WithUsIsGod@yahoo.com

All rights reserved. No parts of this publication may be reproduced or used in any manner whatsoever including stored in a database and/or published in any form or by manner, electronic, mechanical, photocopying, recording or otherwise without the express written permission of the publisher.

Preface

Having a child is one of the most beautiful processes known to mankind. The journey can be bumpy and rough but, the reward is always worthy of the struggle. As I await patiently with much prayer and support, I look forward to spending precious time with my baby girl. Both my husband and I are preparing ourselves to serve as wonderful, cautious and observant parents to our child. We promise to love her unconditionally and protect her as best as we can from the hazards of this world. We pledge to raise her according to God's word, which will provide her with the protection that she will need for the rest of her life. We pray that her arrival be one that is safe, joyous and memorable.

ONE

BACK AGAIN

The Labor and Delivery (L and D) technicians started rolling their eyes whenever they saw me walking up to the triage area. "They could get over themselves. They think they know everything." Even this one judgmental nurse became irritated with me because my blood pressure was so good. It was something close to 100 over 80. Looking at her with disgust, I thought: "So what! I'm still having a headache and my liver enzymes continue to be elevated." All of these healthcare professionals seem to think that I had nothing better to do than to hang out at the hospital. To them, it was as if I enjoyed seeing their precious faces all the time. These people were being very inconsiderate towards me. With an extensive history of birth loss, it was obvious the reason why I was being so cautious and acting moderately anxious. They were behaving like unappreciative females that had only experienced perfect pregnancies. Those fools probably didn't even know what it was like to be in my situation. How dare they judge me! I so desperately wanted to tell them how I felt but, my husband convinced me not to. He didn't want my words to come out the wrong way. He reminded me constantly that: "I didn't know who would deliver the baby." "You can't trust people now a days", he kept saying. "Plus, just be thankful to Jehovah that we've made it this far with so much frustration." Undoubtedly, he was right. I really needed to count my blessings. Hearing him speak those words stopped me from complaining so much and led me to focus more on the current pregnancy.

TWO

BEGINNING

Two years post my ectopic pregnancy, I found myself 29 weeks pregnant with my fourth pregnancy. I could hardly believe it. I was victorious just for getting this far. My husband and I thanked God every day. I could actually feel my baby girl kick and move! It was a great difference from my first pregnancy with Mark-Kenzie. With him, I did not feel anything but gurgling. There was no bumping against my belly, no movements, no kicks! This child exerted more qualities of a normal pregnancy.

On the ultrasounds, she looked just like me. She had huge lips and even bigger eyes. I kept asking my husband: "Do you know anyone in your family who has lips like these?" It was like I was trying to differentiate from one big lip to another. Duh! They were my lips of course. He amused me by answering: "No I can't think of anyone honey." It was quite humorous how we would do that. All in all, I think we were more apprehensive than anything else. These 29 weeks did not come about without many struggles. It took lots of precautions and re-analyzing our situation.

In the very beginning of us trying, we encountered multiple issues. I was so thankful that my husband went and spoke to one of his buddies at work about our fertility problem. It seems that they were just chatting one day and he asked my husband if he had any children. My husband told him: "No and that we were having some trouble in that department." His friend then started explaining the trials him and his wife had recently undergone. He explained how his wife was once pregnant and then in an instance, after a couple of weeks, lost the baby. After that experience, he met someone that told him about an incredible doctor that helped numerous couples get pregnant and successfully have babies. Right then and there, my husband got really excited! He came home that day with big, happy, smiling eyes. It was clear that he had a message to tell. We started talking about the new option and it sounded like a great plan. We desperately wanted to go through with it, so I made an appointment with that doctor's office right away. We prayed on the situation too, hopeful that Jehovah God would guide us through this new process. We felt certain that He would!

THREE
WAITING AND WONDERING

About one month later, I arrived at this special doctor's office for the first time. It wasn't just him though, the office consisted of himself and his associates. The facility was very nice, clean, bright and inviting. The entire staff appeared well put together and knowledgeable. As soon as I walked in and towards the front window, I was asked for all of my information such as identification and health insurance. By this time, I had health insurance from my new job as a psychiatric nurse. This was a job that I hoped to keep for a very long time. Once my documents were returned, I was handed a form to fill out.

As soon as I was done filling out the form and handed it to the receptionist at the front desk, I waited patiently to see the doctor. I felt a little uncomfortable sitting there. The first appointment always seemed to be the longest. Plus, I came right after work and didn't have a chance to freshen up. Yuck! I convinced myself that it was only an initial consultation, so I was okay. There was really no physical assessment completed on the first consultation anyways. It usually is just talking. My main focus was on meeting the doctor. I heard so much about him that I was feeling very excited. I felt like a new kid on the first day of school, ready to embark on new ideas that were never thought to me before.

Amazingly, I never felt hopeless during all of my trials. With all of the miscarriages that occurred, I still felt strong and hopeful. I didn't feel like giving up, not for a third, fourth, fifth, six, 12th or even 50th try: If that many tries were possible. I have heard in the recent pass of doctors shutting down uteruses. Their owners were being told that the organ was wasted and could no longer be utilized. Although, after my prior ectopic pregnancy, my uterus was put on a temporary hiatus. I wanted to make sure that it did not get overused to the point of no repair. I knew how serious an ectopic pregnancy could be to a woman's health in general. If my fallopian tubes would have erupted, I could have easily bled to death. It was possible for me to lose that tube all together, especially since at that time, I was not under the care of a specific physician. To add, a serious condition like an ectopic pregnancy was the last thing I expected. Therefore, until I decided on what I really wanted to do, I found a definitive method to prevent myself from getting pregnant. My fallopian tubes could not handle another shock.

That situation helped me to make a firm decision on whether or not I actually wanted kids. In reality, my husband and I were actually getting old. We were not getting older but old. He was heading towards 36 and I 33. There was no goal of me waiting to that popular age of 35. Call it whatever you want but, starting fertility treatment at those ages was pretty late. It felt like I wasted a good portion of my time being married. We could have been focusing on this very important point and not spending the majority of our moments together dealing with childish nonsense. At some point, it made me think twice about the people around me. "Where were our minds?" The entire situation made me think of whom exactly I had to work with. Thank goodness now, it seemed that we were both thinking straight or at least trying to think straight. There was more positive motivation between the two of us.

FOUR
MY TURN

After a few minutes, one of the techs called my name and I followed her through the door. After my vital signs were obtained, I was escorted to the doctor's office and offered a seat. There, I waited what felt like an eternity. I was beginning to wonder if he had forgotten about me. I'm pretty sure I fell asleep a good portion of the time. I found a cozy chair to put my feet up and kicked back. I was in no mood to bicker, complain or get mad. I used the opportunity to freshen up in the bathroom while waiting. All the while, I was hoping that this doctor did not plan on having a pelvic exam but, only wished to talk. I then rested a bit so that I could have a descent conversation with the doctor about my current medical condition. I wanted to know how he could possibly help me. I still felt excited about meeting him and figured since he was such a popular guy then there was a good reason for his lateness. He may have been busy with other patients.

A few more minutes passed and somebody walked in. I took my feet off of the chair and said hello. It was not at all who I expected to see. It wasn't an older white gentleman like I imagined. Contrary, it was a young white woman, still yapping on her phone as she walked through the door: as if she wasn't already late enough. She looked so young and careless. Giggling to myself, I thought: "She sits down, makes no eye contact and just keeps on talking on that phone." Ridiculous. Nevertheless, I still sat tight patiently and didn't fret. I was still in a good place and nothing was going to get to me. I didn't care about peoples' comportment. I was in the beginning of a very exciting project and exhilaration was in the air, even though I had no idea where this would lead. I was optimism at its best!

FIVE

ADOPTION

At last, the doctor finished talking and turned all of her attention to me. She quickly verified my name and apologized for making me wait so long. Once she evaluated my history, she looked at me and asked: "Have you ever thought about adopting?" This question caught me by surprise. At this stage of attempting to conceive, adoption seemed like a last resort if my husband and I exhausted all of our options. If I had the 50th pregnancy and my uterus was shut down then, I would look into adopting. I still felt young and my mindset was not to care for another person's child. Never did I think of that as an option for myself. Clearly, I was not yet at my wit's end. I was barely at the beginning of trying to get pregnant.

At first, I found it difficult to answer her. I could not comprehend why this woman would ask me such a question. She made me feel even more hopeless! She made me feel as if there was no possible chance of me successfully conceiving and having a child. "Was she getting paid on the side by adoption agencies to make this suggestion?" "What was her real objective?" Sure, I had that ectopic pregnancy, but I prevented any further pregnancies from taking place once I had the IUD (intrauterine device) inserted.

After letting the physician continue to advocate for adoption, I replied with much frustration. I explained that I was not ready to raise someone else's child. I strongly believed that if you have a baby, then you needed to take care of it yourself. That person needed to man up or woman up and care for that child on their own. Plus, I explained to her, that I observed people who adopted children and initially, they looked very unhappy. They actually appeared embarrassed to be seen with the child at first. I further made it clear to her that I was not ready to go through that tough process. I did not feel like having those emotions. After going back and forth for a bit, she stopped badgering me about the subject.

SIX
ACTUAL APPOINTMENT

Once we got down to talking about what mattered to me at that time, I asked about taking aspirin prior to and once I had conceived. I questioned the dosage that I would need to take. I wanted to know about using Lovenox too. "How early would I preferably need to start this blood thinning medication?", I asked. The need to lose weight also came up. I wanted to have a precise plan in place to cover all the bases. There had to be step by step instructions so that no one felt confused on what to do or on what was going on.

As I finished questioning her regarding having a plan in place, the doctor explained to me that she actually would not be going in depth about the pre-conceive planning with me. She apparently would be referring me to a high-risk doctor instead to further discuss the details. Before she could even finish what she was saying, her phone rang and she picked it up. She commenced having another good old conversation with whoever was on the other end. She even gave out another patient's information to the clinician that she was talking to. I guess she figured since I was in uniform, I was under oath and wouldn't say anything. Of course, I didn't care. I was just surprised at her lack of consideration. I wasn't on duty or anything as this was not a practice that I was affiliated with. During her conversation, she even looked at me and told the person that she was talking to: "How great of a client I was and how patient I was behaving." I smiled and shook my head. "I'll take all of the compliments that I can get." Plus, I really didn't care at this point. I was in a good "start-up" mood. Like when a young person is trying to start a new business venture for the first time. Even for the second or the third time. Their excitement cannot be smothered, not by water, smoke, negativity from their surroundings, by rudeness nor by ignorance. They are determined and that was that.

At last, she finished her long conversation and gave me final instructions but, not before giving me her lecture on why I should pick her as my doctor. She was practically begging. It looked as if she was new to the practice and needed clients. She told me that she had 15 years of experience and that she was a good doctor. She made me feel weary and uncomfortable. "Why would a person have to implore a client like that to be her doctor?" I said okay and followed the instructions. I ended up at the receptionist desk for discharge. I got the information to make an appointment with the high-risk doctor and one to see her again.

"Where in the world was that male doctor?" That's who I really came to see. He was the more experienced one and owned the business. I love an old, male doctor. They are so relaxed for many reasons. It could be the old age or the fact that they were male. Whatever it may be, they always seemed very confident, relax and happy. Almost like they have very little stress in their personal lives and in their profession. Maybe I'll request to see him next time. For now, let me just get through the drive home and go to sleep.

SEVEN

UP AGAIN

Waking up from my long, awaited sleep, I saw my husband for the first time that day. He was anxiously waiting to hear about the visit. Of course, he called me before, throughout the day. At those moments, I probably was either busy talking to the doctor, too tired to answer the phone or just passed out sleeping. He would just have to wait till later. Just like me, he too thought I was seeing an old, white, male doctor. That was the picture his friend painted in our minds. Even so, he really wanted to know what the plan was. "How soon could we start trying?" "What medications would I have to be on and for how long?" The list of questions was endless. I explained to him that before we could start any of that, I would have to see the high-risk doctor first. It was important that I had a consultation with that person before anything could be decided.

Upon hearing those words, my husband's eyes looked like they were looking to a far, far, far away future. Like me, he must have thought that I would go to the doctors, comprise a plan and get started on trying right away. Well, unfortunately, it was not that simple. We would have to wait just a little bit longer.

That night I went back to my reality show. I mean "work". Upon coming back home the next day, I set up the appointment to see the high-risk physician. It seemed easy enough, until they requested information about past pregnancies and past medical records. Now the fun part begins. I had to get those papers from three different hospitals. Let's see how much enjoyment I would get out of this.

EIGHT

RACING

As I grasped the task of retrieving that information, I realized how difficult it would be to retrieve all of those documents. For starter, I tried making phone calls to see if that would get the process rolling along. It was like hitting a brick wall. Those phone calls brought no result. All that I got was that I needed to go directly to each location. To add, none of the sites were within the hospital limits. I had to go and sign release paperwork to have the information either faxed over to the high-risk doctor or given to me to give to the doctor in person. Plus, for some of the facilities, I had to pay if I chose to have the documents handed straight to me. One hospital gave me such a hard time that I remembered sitting in my car crying out of frustration. I just wanted the stupid records in my hands. I only wanted to hand them to the doctor so that I could get started with this baby making process. If I didn't have all of the paperwork, I couldn't see the high-risk doctor. I couldn't receive the all so important consultation that I needed.

That same day, I walked myself to the record department and requested they give me all my medical records right away! The receptionist asked from what date to what date. I told her that I needed all of my records and that I did not have any dates. She looked suspicious at me and asked: "What was it for?" That was when I started to get upset. "None of your business", I thought. "I need them so I could give them to another doctor." "What was it to her! They were my records! I could request them whenever I pleased!" She continued to give me a hard time. I prepared to give her a tough time too. It looked like her manager or supervisor was right in the back and paying attention to what was happening. She herself looked scared and suspicious. It dawned on me later on that maybe they thought that I was filing a lawsuit and that was the reason I needed all of the information at once. After a little bit of a struggle though, she handed me all of my paperwork.

"Thank God I didn't lose my cool." Now I could go to sleep knowing that I got all the information. I could rest knowing that I didn't have to push the appointment back any further. Lord knows we did not want to do that.

NINE

WEIGHT LOSS

The appointment with the high-risk doctor was quite a distance away. It was scheduled for approximately one month. In the mean time, I had some work to get started on. I needed to get a good weight loss program in place. I couldn't just focus on losing the extra fat that I carried around but, on becoming healthy. I needed to eat a good variety of food. It was dire that I consumed nutrient filled foods that would make my body more conducive to conceiving and growing a healthy baby. I aimed to eat food that would replenish my body and not just fill it. My objective was to clean out my system. In a sense I would rid my body of all impurities and toxins. No caffeine, no alcohol, no medications that might greatly affect my health would touch my lips. I even planned to stop drinking certain types of tea that might inadvertently be causing dehydration. Anything that caused difficulties conceiving and carrying a child, had to go.

The process started promptly, as I was running out of time. I immediately started taking my daily 325 milligrams (mg) of Aspirin as I was supposed to have been doing before anyways. Some weight came off from having started to work out post my ectopic pregnancy but, it felt like I was watching my caloric intake a bit too strictly. That diet was rigid and would not last long term. To add, it felt like those extra pounds that were loss were mostly water weight. I needed to focus on eating healthy foods such as kale, collard greens, spinach and broccoli. Drinking plenty of water and exercising daily would also aid the routine. Basically, I planned to start a long-term regimen that I could follow for the rest of my life. That was a goal worth setting! If I am successful at having one baby, I might think about having a few more.

"It's all about finding the secret." Once you know what works for you, then you have mastered how to successfully conceive and have a baby. You now know what works for your situation and what you needed to do before going through the process. Both my husband and I hoped that would happen to us. He would joke: "You're about to have 10 to 12 kids", "We're going to have a little soccer team." That was so cute of him.

The funny thing was, that exact scenario could actually be a possibility since both our families had a history of multiples. My own grandmother had 10 children. Her cousin had eight and that was after having great difficulties conceiving and experiencing many pregnancy losses herself. She traveled all over Haiti in search of a good doctor. Once she found that person, there was no stopping her and her husband. Then there was my husband's uncle who had 12 children. Absolutely, this was in our blood! It was definitely a possibility. I don't imagine myself getting upset if that fantasy came true either. I do believe that my husband and I would be thrilled and delighted. The only problem was, we would need a whole lot more money. Plus, I would not want to live in the house that we live in now. We would need to get a bigger place. Silly us, we hadn't even had one child nor had we gone through the initial steps. Now, we were both seriously thinking about having a football team. Funny! There's no harm in dreaming though. There was no harm in fantasizing and imagining. We could have fun with our situation. Infertility couldn't take that away from us.

At the gym, I told the instructor what my weight loss goals were and what for. I decided to just be honest and tell her that I was trying to have a baby. I felt comfortable enough woman to woman. She was encouraging at first, then when she started examining my body, she could see that I was pregnant before. The shape of my abdomen on the computer analysis graph they used made it very clear. Once she noted that, her facial expression automatically changed. At first, she was talking about her own child and appreciating what God gave her. Then she started acting very uncomfortable. She realized that the most amount of fat focused in my belly had to be caused by pregnancy. It definitely couldn't have been a beer gut. Even I was surprised to see the image. There was nothing you could hide from those computer graphs. Although I personally felt slimmer, those graphical images did not lie! To make matters worse, viewing the images changed how the lady acted.

Here we go again! The pity party was on full speed. The lady almost couldn't finish assessing me. I thought she was going to break down and cry. It's so annoying to me when people do that. I do not feel pity for myself. I may feel sad or confused about the situation but, not pitiful or hopeless. At times, I had some difficulties coming to term with the situation and why I was suffering through it. I couldn't always image the next step because I just wanted to have everything happen naturally and spontaneously. I never felt sorry for myself though. I always bounced back to my cheerful self.

Now for this trainer who was acting like a fool. "Forget her! How dare she make me feel uncomfortable! Doesn't she realize that acting like that only affects me in a negative way? Doesn't she realize how uneasy she makes me feel?" I hurried up and finished the assessment so I could get out from her sight. By the end, this lady couldn't even look me in the eyes. I thought that she was about to cry. "Man, she really needed to pull herself together." I myself didn't even feel that uncomfortable and it was my situation.

With high confidence, I still took some of her courses. Despite the fact that she continued to have a hard time looking straight at me, I stayed on my weight loss journey. The whole reaction seemed comical to me. I couldn't help but to laugh at her. Ironically, I had pity for her and not the other way around. She needed to relax and just drop it. I was going to be fine. In my heart, I believed that I was going to make it. Yes! I was going to reach my objective. With plenty of help, I was going to reach it!

TEN

HEALTH REGIMEN CONTINUE

So on with the rigorous boot camp exercises. I went at least twice, often three times a week. There were different trainers that taught the classes. I felt exhausted after doing squat-thrusts, sit-ups, crunches, jumping jacks, weight lifting and all that mess. With all of this work, I was expecting to get great results, fast!

I continued measuring my food to get accurate amounts but, I did not enslave myself to doing that. I ate oat to replace the heavy amount of carb filled rice that us Caribbean folks loved to eat and I continued drinking plenty of water. "Oh how I looked forward to weighting myself to see how much I had loss!" I felt positive that it was a good deal of pounds. "With all of that work, I was certain that I would see some results."

The first thing that I did upon arriving at the gym, was step onto the scale to see my progress. To my surprise, I had gained weight. The opposite happened! "Could it be all muscle gain?", I tried to convince myself. I was, after all, lifting weight to help my body lose fat quicker. That's what all of the trainers always suggested. "Lift weight to lose more fat. Gain more muscle mass to help burn fat faster", they all said. Indeed, gaining more muscle mass did aid in burning fat quicker and easier. It seemed that it was a time taking process, though. I don't think that I had that much time on my hands. For some reason, this was not working for me. I needed to see results faster! I was not training for a weight lifting competition nor training to be a body builder.

Just then, I remembered a coworker of mines had mentioned that her daughter loss a great deal of weight by walking and jogging. She said that weight lifting should be done way later in a weight loss program not at the beginning. "Now why didn't I think of that?" I had plenty of exercise (digital video disc) DVDs at home that focused on walking to lose weight. I used them to help me lose 50 pounds in prior years. I kept those DVDs as back up in case I preferred to walk inside instead. So, digging through my old stuff I went.

ELEVEN

OTHER METHOD

Around my neighborhood was perfect for walking and jogging. I made the decision to walk outdoors to start. There was plenty of other people that did that too near where I lived. I felt safe and comfortable enough to walk by myself. Plus, I felt I knew the neighborhood pretty well. I would go as far as three or four blocks up. The good thing was that the blocks were long, so I got a really good workout. Everything was going perfectly. I felt energetic and had even started to see results within a matter of weeks. I believe maybe about five pounds weight loss was observed. Everything was fabulous until one day.

One evening, I went for my walk a little later than usual. It was about six o'clock at night but, the sun was still out. I decided to quickly go for my routine stroll. I went up four long blocks to the popular gas station, went in and got some free ice and water and came back out. I only stayed there for about five minutes and then headed back. On my way home, I felt somebody following me. He looked like a very mentally unstable individual. I decided to cross the street to avoid him. There was a laundromat there. I was going to try to wait him out or call my husband to pick me up.

As soon as I tried to cross, he too tried to cross. I tried walking down the block, he tried walking as well. So, finally I just stood there with my arms crossed staring at him. As if to say: "Well what do you want to do." I did not keep on walking. There were trees further down and he could really attack me without anyone ever seeing anything. But right where I was standing, there was enough light for someone to see. A few seconds later, he ran across the street. I think I confused him. Plus, I was looking at a car parked near us with someone in it. That guy was really weird. I didn't even have anything in my hands. I only had a free ice and water but, threw away the cup when I was done. Scary! That could have been some pervert or a murderer. God really was with me that evening. I quickly walked back home. From that day on, I was very careful not to go out too late at night. The neighborhood was not as safe as I thought. As a matter of fact, from that point on, I ended up going to the gym to walk on the treadmill. I still walked around the neighborhood but, only in broad daylight. I was not about to let darkness find me out there anymore.

To help keep track of my progress, I downloaded a step counting (application) APP on my phone to help me track how much I walked for that day. It helped me to keep track of the number of calories I burned each day too. I even had an APP that calculated all of the food that I ate every day. It added up the calories from fat, carbs and protein while differentiating how much of each I consumed that particular day. This helped me to determine which food to eat that were healthiest. Now I felt like I was getting result! I felt light too. Actually, I felt amazing! I think it was the energy I was getting from walking all the time.

TWELVE

WORK

At work, I was having another kind of fun. I was enjoying getting used to my new job. It looked like something that I would love to do long term. I did not mind the patients at all. They were actually the least of my problems. The patients acted like they had sense. They knew that they were there to get help. It was the employer and employees who were the headaches. Those individuals acted like complete animals. They made the job 5000 times harder than it really was. In reality, all I had to do was complete a few paperwork and keep the patients safe at night. But oh no, some techs (technicians) wanted to make that simple task difficult. It was so sad how these jokers could make an easy job like that seem so tough. They were out to ruin it for everyone!

Dealing with my coworkers was something amazing! They made that psychiatric facility to be more like a reality television show. Attitude, neck snapping and hand waving was always in play. People went into work to outdo their selves each shift. It turned into a big competition. No one really came to work, they came to join the show. The rumor roaming around was that the new boss fired all the old workers that threatened a union and hired brand new ones. He somehow made sure all of those people vanished. It was something like a great disappearing act. The complaint all around was: "How could he fire someone that has worked here for thirty plus years? How can somebody just do that?" Either that or they would complain. They would say: "He just fired that worker because he did he's job too good." The grumble was endless. According to those that were familiar with the situation, people were indeed getting fired left and right for no apparent reason. Evidently, there was more to their discharges. Plus, you would think that those that remained and had observed all these people get dismissed would be acting differently. At the very least they would be showing some kind of respect for the job. To my dismay, that was not the case.

One day, while walking into work, behaving as politely as I possibly could, a male coworker decided that he would be unpleasant towards me that shift. As I was saying hello to everyone, this old man starts barking at me exclaiming how much he hated working with me. The announcement came as a complete shock to me since the night before, we were as nice as we could be with each other. I figured, he must have had a bad day and decided to take it out on little old me. His aim for the night was to act as nasty as he could act. To make matters worse, this individual called himself a "man of God." He upsetted me so much that night that I wanted to cry. The very least, I felt embarrassed. Certainly, I was not going to return his nasty attitude, it was not in me to do that. "If he wanted to give me a hard way to go, then that was on him." "He could be the rotten egg amongst us, not I."

Another long-time worker decided he wanted to sabotage me too. I'll call him "Mr. Backstabber for no reason." He proved to be a real idiot. After having worked with him for a few nights, I thought very highly him. I enjoyed working with him and had nothing but positive words to say about the man. One day I call up to another floor and he answered. I was happy to hear his voice. I said hello and he rudely responded. I assumed that he was having a bad night. It was, after all, a psych (psychiatric) hospital and things could happen that frustrate the mess out of you. Later, after not seeing him for a while, I asked about him and it turned out that he was not only the biggest backstabber but the stupidest backstabber. Apparently, he went to upper management and reported me, stating that "I was not doing my job." He even dared them to confirm by looking at the cameras that were installed at every corner. Unfortunately for him, upper management did just that. They looked at the cameras and the cameras told the truth. As it turned out, it was him they found not doing his job and so immediately, they fired him.

I never even knew about the ordeal. I was actually concerned for his well-being and that was the reason I asked for him. I thought maybe as an old veteran he might have gotten sick. In reality, he was sick alright. He had the devil in him. And you know what the devil can do to you. He can make you play your own self. As a woman of God, He has always protected me. Maybe that old man didn't know me long enough to know that.

To make matters worse, as veterans of the job, those older workers were setting such a terrible example for the younger employees. The new crew that they hired soaked up all the negative behavior like a sponge. The place became one big playground. The new staff was disgusting, to say the least. One technician became violently upset whenever I asked her the simplest question. If I just asked, "What was that patient's blood pressure?", she started moving her body angrily, like a rabid dog. She looked so ugly doing it too. She proved to have no class and no self-respect. She reminded me of those women on the reality television shows that fought like animals for money. They were the newer version of slavery and that's what the younger workers loved to imitate. At times, I wondered if any of them had ever actually worked a real job before. This behavior became the main reason other staff members started exiting like high speed race cars. No one was staying at that job. Everyone that came, gave it a go and said no. Ironically, all of those people had the same reason for quitting. "Staffing was horrible!" The workers were rude, obnoxious and disrespectful.

Despite agreeing one hundred percent with those that left, I decided to stay. I for one, enjoyed working with my patient population. It was way less extensive than my prior job as a trauma nurse. I found his job to be not only repetitive but, laid back. There was always the risk of injuring yourself dealing with a psych patient but, that was a part of every nursing position. You really couldn't win with this career. As for me, I was determined to hang in there because I really needed the health insurance, which I believed was far more superior than that of the government. So, I decided to stick it out despite all of the nonsense.

THIRTEEN

HIGH-RISK

It was finally time for my very special, exciting and life changing appointment! I knew they had all of the papers they needed. I especially went and dropped off one copy myself. I didn't have it faxed or forwarded, I delivered it myself hand to hand. Now the time had finally come. My husband and I waited patiently in the high-risk doctor's sitting area until we were called. After a few minutes, we finally got to see the doctor. She was an adorable, little, short, red headed woman. She looked like those cute Irish performers. Her long pointy nose was as red as her cheeks. Her entire appearance would make her the star of a show. All she needed was a little green hat. I couldn't wait to hear what she had to say.

We sat down with her and explained what we wanted. We told her that we wanted to have a baby. She asked a list of questions about my past medical history and prior pregnancies. She also asked about both our family history; if there were any medical issues and birth defects. She questioned regarding family members from my mother's side and from my father's side. Likewise, for my husband, the doctor questioned the history from his mother's side and from his father's side. Very extensive was the interview. She then asked if I was currently taking my oral anticoagulants. I told her yes but that I could be noncompliant at times. She gave me a really stern look with that response. It basically meant for me to get it together.

We then discussed how many milligrams of my Aspirin I was presently taking and how much I should switch to once I became pregnant. She told me that there were new studies that showed that pregnant women could take two 'baby aspirins' instead of one. Since I had been aware of the one 81 mg of Aspirin for years, I opted to stay with that amount. We continued our conversation with weight loss, healthy diet plan and exercise. We spoke of blood thinning injections to take once pregnant and how much dosage was necessary. I asked her about prenatal vitamins, but she only focused on Folic Acid. She didn't give me a prescription for it but, told me to get 1000 mg of the supplement from a local vitamin store. When we asked what my husband should do, she replied: "Nothing." There was nothing that he needed to do other than get the deed done right. I was the one that needed to care for my body as well as possible. The whole thing basically fell on me, the female.

Right after the consultation, my husband and I went straight to our local pharmacy to purchase all of the required items. We got a bottle 325mg of Aspirin to make sure I never ran out and then searched for the 1000mg of Folic Acid that we could only find at a local, brand-name vitamin store. Immediately, I started taking both medications. Despite the High-risk doctor telling us that my husband did not need to do anything, he still started focusing more on his health. He contacted his friend that referred the associates of doctors in the first place and asked about what regimen he followed before producing their beautiful baby girl and received some great tips. We were now feeling optimistic about our situation!

FOURTEEN
WAITING

Staying on top of my doctors' appointments was not easy but, I made it my main priority. At some point, I even went and got another physician's opinion just to be on the safe side. I would have contacted my doctor from my previous stillbirth but, encountered such a hard time reaching them. It was not clear to me why I had such difficulties reaching that office. Hence, I went to see another specialist from a near reputable hospital. We sat and spoke together about my current and past situation as I had done with numerous other professionals. Like most physicians, she seemed scared of my history. She was young in appearance and didn't really want to be bothered with me. When I asked her about using anticoagulants, she became defensive, like someone that was ready to fight. At some point, she even looked petrified! Finally, she suggested that I go to another professional if I deemed fit. She clearly wanted to relieve herself of me: the miracle patient that scared every physician in town. I am sure that they all wondered, "How is she still here?" "How on earth was she still walking around?"

Healthcare could be very risky business, especially with patients like me. Sometimes, not getting a patient is far better than having to deal with risking your license and reputation. I certainly could understand why she didn't want to deal with me.

Having to deal with someone who had a history like myself, with the risk of possible grand mal seizure during her last pregnancy would not be easy. In addition, I was obese, had high cholesterol, poor circulation and poor past family medical history. If I saw me walking towards me, I would run away too. The doctor that I was seeing now was perfect for me. Sure, I wasn't actually seeing him at the time but, it was still his business. It was members of his team that were treating me. I felt more confident that I was in good hands after speaking to this young girl. The only problem was, I've yet to see those hands. It was impertinent for me to meet this doctor, the man in charge before I trusted my life to his practice. I kindly took the hints from the young lady in front of me and headed on my way.

FIFTEEN

RE-DO

At home, we were getting our bathroom remodeled. We were referred to a general contractor by our friends to do the job. The guy seemed pretty well skilled. We felt confident that he would deliver good result. We saw his work at a friend's basement that he remodeled. It was well done with a few finishing touches left untidy. He did it at a low price so, we opted to see what he would deliver.

Upon his initial evaluation he tried eagerly to influence me to get only a slitter of tile decoration mounted on the wall. He aimed to make me think it was the style now-a-day. He debated that everyone did their bathrooms the same way. I didn't buy it. Plus, I wasn't trying to be like everybody else. I figured, if I'm going to remodel my bathroom then I'm going to remodel in every sense of the word. I wanted something that stood out; something that was different from everybody else's. The style had to be one that everyone could wow over once they saw it. That bathroom had to be something that no one had ever seen before. I wanted artistic designs, beautiful colors, unique structures and antiquity. Most of all, it had to be full of beautiful ceramic tiles from top to bottom. In my mind, I was living in a museum and even in the bathroom, I was to be mesmerized.

I purchased base tiles of cream color. Then, for the main attraction, artistic ceramic tiled mural of a gorgeous floral design with matte finish were specially ordered. The mural consisted of beautiful red and pink roses draping over an antique, gold vase. The rich, vibrant, colors made the painting come to life. I even ordered eight matching accent tiles to have scattered throughout. Truly, they were not just ceramic tiles or collage to me. I felt that I was experiencing the creation of a highly skilled artist. I could barely control myself. My mouth drooled and I could almost smell the sweetness of those roses. Truth is, both my husband and I could barely control ourselves.

During the renovation, my husband gave me full creative control. He didn't even bother going to the store with the contractor to buy the materials. He stayed behind to get the bathroom ready for construction. He told the contractor that I was the boss and that he wanted no parts of it. The guys were chuckling to themselves. They couldn't get enough of him. I was glad that he gave me that power. As an artistic and meticulous woman, I liked knowing everything that was taking place. This was the more so true when it came to redesigning any part of the house. This project really was something to get us through our current situation. The hump of waiting for this baby making process to start and take effect, would not be easy to climb.

In the meanwhile, life continued. My husband and I spoke of our plans. He remained on top of all my doctor's appointments. One day, out of the blue, he questioned exactly which doctor I met the very first time I visited the office. Right then and there, we decided that we really wanted to meet the man in charge. We wanted to certify how this office operated and make sure everyone was on the same train.

One phone call to the office, and we changed the appointment to see him instead.

SIXTEEN

MORE LABOR

I was starting to get use to my new job. Honestly, I enjoyed going there minus the troublesome co-workers. The only thing that I did not appreciate was working five nights a week straight and the being on call whatever weekend they wanted me to be available. No advance notice was ever given either. The manager would sometimes slack and not inform staff members of their scheduled on-call weekends. Later, she would try to threaten whoever did not show up.

One weekend, I had a prearrangement and was out of state. I had no idea that I was on-call for that particular weekend. No one had informed me and there wasn't any paperwork provided either. Obviously, I was unavailable to work that night. So, I did the one thing that I could do and didn't bother answering the phone when they called. The next night, I spoke to the supervisor and she said that the same scenario was happening every weekend. People were not being notified ahead of time of their weekends to work and thus causing the facility to always be short on the weekends. "Well, especially on the weekends, they were always short the other days too."

Another Saturday, I actually came in thinking it was my weekend to work since I received a phone call telling me so. From the moment I walked in to work, it was trouble. For starters, I didn't work on my usual floor. I got pulled to a totally different floor. That unit was a more aggressive environment than I was use to working in. That unit was for intense adults, not for sweet older adults like I was accustomed to working with. These patients we're young men and women with history of heavy drug abuse and as the name indicated, they tended to get extremely violent. It was clear that I wasn't swimming with the dolphins anymore, I was spinning with the sharks. "Hopefully this would be a quick night and I could go home and go to sleep." It was never easy working on a floor you're not familiar with.

To make matters worse, I was working with a completely different set of staff members. I had never seen these group of people before. It was not difficult to imagine how some of them reacted. "Those cruel, adult, professionals" acted like anything but. They managed to get lose like kids do when a substitute teacher takes over. From childhood to adulthood, those personalities managed to stay the same. I tried my best to ignore the nonsense and made my rounds with all of my checks. A few hours later, we got some admissions and that was when all went downhill. The one female technician started acting out. She created a reason not to help the patient, making matters bad for everyone else. I knew I saw her eyeing me the moment I came in. That look was no surprise to me. It said: "This black girl is younger than me and has a degree, why can't I do the same." She started making comments demeaning her own position as if to show that she had no responsibility towards the patients and everything fell on me. At the end, she had the nerve to call the supervisor on me and complain. I knew right then and there that I would not be coming back the next day. I would find a way out of this.

The moment that I got home, I double checked the list for nurses that were supposed to be on call that weekend and realized that my name was not on for that particular weekend after all. Saved again! I had answered that phone call without even verifying. Now, for certain, I was not at work that next day. Never mind the manager who messed that up again! I was not about to make any more sacrifices that I didn't have to make, not in my current medical state. I did not need the extra stress!

SEVENTEEN

APPOINTMENT

That Monday, my husband and I both went to see the doctor in charge. Just like before, we waited patiently until my name was called. Then we were escorted to his office. Obviously, he had the better, bigger room. There was a window and everything. A nice dark, cherry wood desk almost the size of a dining room table, took up most of the space. We sat waiting for a bit and then popped in an interesting looking man. He was a complete contrast to the prior physician that saw me last, by all means. This physician had a nasty, filthy medical coat that looked like it hadn't been washed in years. I couldn't decipher if he worked in a coal mine or saw female patients for a living. I didn't detect any odor so, I figured it was just stained and not actually soiled. I couldn't be one hundred percent sure though. His expression showed that he could care less about his appearance. He certainly was confident in that trifling get-up. Tall, blonde as we expected with old age written all over his face. He proved to be very relaxed, maybe a bit too relaxed. My only prayers were that he never physically examined me with that disgusting coat on. Yuck! I might leave with bumps and puss all over. I most likely wouldn't even be able to determine where what came from. It seemed that "white" coat had a little something from everyone. Thank goodness that room wasn't made for physical examination anyways. Let the verbal consultation begin!

We sat and talked for a while and considered different options for prenatal and postnatal care. We decided on weight loss goals and need for strict regimen of all anticoagulants and medications ordered. After careful examination of my records and a quick verbal assessment of my husband, he sent both of us to get lab work drawn. He was quick and swift; just as I expected from a man of his stature. He wasted no time on his part.

Post the assessment, we thought that maybe he would keep me as his patient but, he referred me back to that other doctor. I wasn't surprised. He probably just kept the easier files. No sense in messing with this difficult patient, not at this stage in his career. He could do without the extra stress, I was sure. Upon leaving, I almost didn't want to shake his hand. I mean, I love laidback doctors as much as the next person but, his appearance could use a little freshening up. My only hopes were that the massive amount of discolorations were ink and other non-washable, non-bodily residue. That's the best explanation I could think of.

The lab works were obtained, even though we had no idea what they were. For some reason, I neglected to ask. I do recall they were general lab like CBC (complete blood count) and BMP (basic metabolic panel). Since I knew that someone would call with the results, I didn't feel concerned about knowing at the current time. The little set up that they had was very nice. As soon as a patient was finished seeing the doctor, they simply went and got their blood drawn. I liked that very much! It was less of a hustle than having to take time out to get blood work at another facility. Compliments to them on the convenience to clients.

EIGHTEEN

NEXT STEP

Approximately three months had passed since all of the consultations and doctor's visits commenced. Now, we felt prepared to get the ball rolling. I was over zealous to start. I could hardly wait another second, let along another day or month. I just wanted that IUD out of me so that my husband and I could get busy working on our new project. I notified my physician and asked if I could have the IUD taken out? For about three months, I had been taking all of my medications regularly. In addition, I purchased a multivitamin with 1000mg folic acid and iron in it. It perplexed me as to why the high-risk physician did not prescribed that in the first place. Plus, my primary doctor said that all women, whether attempting to bear a child or not, should be taking prenatal vitamins daily. Its essential to every women's general health. Especially now that they were over the counter with no prescription required. The chief OBGYN (Obstetrician/Gynecologist) wasn't quite sure if I should start trying or not. He wanted to run some more test on me. He told my husband and I to make an appointment to discuss further our options and that's what we did.

On the next appointment, I basically had my lab drawn. He ordered a CBC and a BMP to check all of my levels such as kidney functions and hemoglobin. Once the results came back, I was cleared to have the IUD taken out. He just wanted to make sure my medication regimen was working. It was time to remove that device!

I arrived promptly at another one of his office, knowing that my female doctor would not be available to perform the procedure. My only option was to have dear older, male doctor complete the process. This crazy looking man was the one to have me lay down and pull that device out of my cervical cavity. With his expertise usually came that nasty coat though. I guess I had no choice.

When I got there, I actually did not remember what the man had on. One thing I knew was if he had that coat on, I would have noticed and remembered. I only recalled laying back and spreading those legs wide. After a few minutes of digging, he waved the gooey prize up in the air full of mucous. It was out! Time to get busy!

Before I left that day, we talked about delivery locations and options. I wanted to know where exactly did he and his team deliver. Plus, I wanted to know if he had ever worked or was familiar with treating patients that did not accept blood. That was an important factor for me. As soon as he heard that mentioned, he appeared to really hesitate; so much so that he scared me. Maybe he was uncomfortable with the procedures that the program entailed. He had me thinking that perhaps he had some prior issues with bloodless medicine patients. Nevertheless, I still left my power of attorney with him, in my file that depicted what I wished to be done in certain emergency situations. He ordered me an extra dose of 1000mg folic acid and I went home to rethink what was right for me to do.

NINETEEN

NEW MD

Something was not adding up. I was wondering about different events that took place at that doctor's office. To start, the female doctor that I first saw had me feeling suspicious. She practically begged me to be her patient. She acted as if she was not a competent doctor. Then, whenever I would go to the front office, there was a great deal of uneasiness from the staff members regarding her. Once, I specified that she was my doctor and one lady became very much in shock. She had her eyes opened wide appearing to be in disbelief, as if to say "oh goodness no!" Another time, while at the window handling my discharge, an older lady literally shook her head "no". I had to shadily check all around me to see if anyone else was observing this. When I looked back at her, she shook her head side to side "no" once again. If those weren't enough clues then, I didn't know what was. Basically, those women were telling me not to choose that particular doctor. For whatever reasons, the warning signs were there.

The primary doctor, although very skilled, worried me as well. He seemed quite uncomfortable working with the bloodless methods that I proposed through my durable power of attorney. I felt skeptical and decided to go somewhere else. It was important that I went to a hospital that specialized in bloodless medicine and one that I was already accustomed to.

Once I finally met with my old doctors after many failed attempts at making an appointment, I sat down and spoke to her about the plan that was already made. She seemed somewhat upset and disappointed that I didn't contact her first. I explained to her that the other doctor had a high-risk physician on board. She became even more upset and exclaimed, "so do we." "Oh well", I thought.

"Maybe if it was easier to make an appointment with your lazy receptionist, I would have gone to you first." Anyhow, I was here now and that's what mattered. I hoped to enjoy my stay with her and her colleagues. I knew she was a highly recommended physician but, she was already starting to pester me. Maybe it was my anxiousness to start trying for a baby. Either way, it seemed that something had changed about her. She appeared to be under a lot more stress.

TWENTY

AT LAST

At last, we could start trying to conceiving! Fun times were here! My husband and I enjoyed the opportunity presented to us immensely. It got so ridiculous, that I would sometimes be laying in bed during the day and call on my husband to come make sweet love to me. It felt like a movie or some hot romance novel. We would kiss and hold each other afterwards, knowing the purpose of our union that very moment. We would chat about a possible future with children. Discussing names and travel plans with our kids had become common amongst us.

Then, there were times when the love making got to feel like work. It became tiresome, if you can believe that. We would be forced to be all over each other and have intercourse. I would be tired and wanting to be asleep after work but, would have to wait around for my husband to come home during his break. We weren't aware of when to have sex, so we made sure we covered all fields. It got to a point that I wanted to go to sleep in the middle of it all. Not even in my dreams did I want to be that sexually active. My husband started complaining saying, "People in the streets get pregnant faster than this." I had to keep reminding him that we weren't "street people." We were civilized, true Christians. Plus, many other couples had the same issue. We weren't the only ones going through this. We were not alone in this situation but, we had to be patient in order to see results.

After one month of trying, that's exactly what happened. I took a pregnancy test and it was positive! I was pregnant! "Well, that was easy enough." I became so excited and called my doctor right away to let her know. Promptly, I made an appointment to get an ultrasound and start my Lovenox. Then, still feeling elated, I went to the gym and walked on a treadmill. I felt so great and at that time, the gym was the only place that I wanted to be. One week later, after telling my boss and the night supervisor, I started bleeding. I bled for what was about two weeks straight. Silly thing is, my stomach had started to show even at one month pregnant due to my prior pregnancies. I was excitingly pushing it out, making was not apparent noticeable. By the time those two weeks were over, they could look at my stomach and see that I had miscarried. The difference was so obvious.

Despite this loss, my spirit wasn't down though. I still felt motivated to keep trying. In all reality, it was only the first time that we technically ever tried. All of our prior pregnancies were accidental. No intended effort was ever made at those times. There was no prepping completed so, I reasoned positively with myself that I really had only failed once and could stand to try again.

For my husband though, it was an entirely different story. This man was crushed, hurt, upset, discouraged and bitter. All of the negative emotions you could think of, he had. Our expression of emotion was night and day, hot and cold. We were at total opposite ends of the Earth. He became angry like he had lost a bar fight. His veins popped like a silver back gorilla ready to charge. I had to calm him down. "This is our first time really trying", I reminded him. "We're only in the beginning phase of this journey, let's not give up so soon." Eventually, the little pep talk got to him and we took a breather until we figured out what we wanted to do next.

TWENTY-ONE
STARTING AGAIN

Meanwhile, at work things were not looking up. This group of employees were more than just rude or incompetent, they were violent. I had never in my years working, met such a staff. The environment was like a reality television series that had train wrecked and was hard to watch. It really was the most out of control experience that I ever had. I was happy to find out that I was not the only one who felt that way. A large number of people continued to quit. They all had the same reasons for leaving: "Poor staffing!" It wasn't that staffing was necessarily poor in quantity, which it was, but in quality too.

One nurse even burst into tears at how horrible some of the staff members had been treating her. They would yell at her, switch assignments, and act disrespectful towards her whenever they pleased. After handing in her two weeks letter of resignation, she would look so depressed coming into work. She could not keep her composure. Sometimes, she would start to cry in between sentences at the thought of how she was mistreated. It was an odd sight to see. This grown woman had only been at the job for a couple of months; that was less time than I worked there. Already, she was broken down so badly by these ratchet employees that she was reduced to tearing up as if someone close to her had died and she was grief-stricken. This woman hated it there with a vengeance. I felt bad for her but, happy at the same time that someone else had the same feelings that I did. These events gave weight to any complaints I would later have or any grievances that could come against me.

One day, as I was on my way out, a male coworker decided that he wanted to treat me like his footstool. He started 'pushing' me around like I was less than an animal. I quickly removed myself from near him and finished giving report. The other two staff members present attempted to speak up but, I was in no mood to argue all the time with grown adults. My objective at that exact moment was to finish report and go home and go to sleep. With the ridiculous tolerance of the management team at that facility, that man could have thrown me across a room and still have 'higher up' try to sugar coat the incident.

After many equivalent incidents, I decided to do something about the problem. One day, after work, I went and emailed management and later reported the entire incident to human resources for my record's sake. Certainly, I did not believe that anything serious would be done and it wasn't.

The work place violence there was incredible! The entire scene or atmosphere of that place was intolerable to say the least. You would think that it was a "ma and pa" operation, just starting out. You would not imagine that this company was a huge corporation spread throughout the entire United States. They really needed to clean up their act.

TWENTY-TWO
WHAT NEXT

After our most recent miscarriage, both my husband and I were in a much better mood. We were ready to get back on that horse and start riding again. This time we weren't going to stop until we reached our final destination. We planned to be successful! "No playing games down this rugged road."

First thing first, I taught myself how to calculate an ovulation schedule. We aimed to have intercourse at the best possible time to produce a well, fertilized egg. I continued taking all of my medications and eating right. I even kept exercising but, this turn around, not so vigorously. I mostly did my walking around the block during daytime, when everyone else was out. In addition, I very closely monitored my daily steps and nutritional intake. I had a great balance on the whole regimen.

At some point, I felt that my weight loss had ceased. To help, I incorporated another special tool, fasting. I heard mentioned once of a group of people breaking their fast early in the morning. It was at that moment that I understood the word "breakfast" to have a totally different meaning. I had never understood it that way before to mean break a fast. It all made sense though. A normal person is not supposed to eat during the night. A healthy body needs to rest at night, not gorge any kind of food. Ever since then, I took fasting as a healthy alternative. I began to cut down my food consumption while I worked at night little by little until I could stand not to eat at all. If I did feel hungry, I would fill myself up with plenty of water. If that failed and I found myself needing more energy, which I rarely did, I brought along some raw vegetables to munch on. All in all, this way of thinking began to help me achieve my goals faster.

About a month later, while on a mini vacation, I suspected

pregnancy. My menstrual period came and stayed for a very long time. That, I knew, was a clear sign of having conceived. It was even more clear than the prior pregnancy, for I didn't recall having an extended period like I was having now. Whenever that happened, it gave the feeling that the body was cleaning or ridding itself of all impurities. The body was freeing itself of any kind of interference that could interrupt the attachment and growth of the newly formed embryo. It honestly felt like a natural detoxification. The body apparently had its own way of keeping itself clean and healthy. This time, I put myself on an unofficial bedrest. The job had become way too risky for me so, I asked for some time off. In the back of my mind, I wondered if I would ever go back. Besides having terrible co-workers, there were very little safety mechanisms in place at the facility itself. One month later, my period didn't come and I took a pregnancy test. It was positive! I get excited every time, no matter what the outcome may be.

TWENTY-THREE
FIRST THING

It was thrilling, once again, to find out that I was expecting! The first thing that I did was call my doctor. I made an appointment to see her and asked to have an ultrasound (US) done that same day. As the days and weeks progressed, I called back numerous times to confirm that appointment and those instructions. Once I arrived to the office, I double checked that the ultrasound was ordered. No surprise! I was met with much hesitation. I figured there would be an issue since the stupid scheduler sounded reluctant every time I spoke to her on the phone. Whatever happened though, I had better be getting an ultrasound that same day. If not, it was going to be a major problem.

Once I saw the doctor, she acted as if she wasn't going to order the test. She looked like she had no intentions at all. I couldn't start my injectable anticoagulants unless I had an ultrasound to assure the baby was in the right place. What was the big deal! I didn't get pregnant by accident, there was a plan in place. She proceeded to do a full body exam, as if that meant something to me. I pretty much told her: "I'm not leaving until I got the procedure done and my medication started immediately." I was seriously ready to say something in a form of document. "How grumpy and impatient I had become in the past years." Again, with this stupid scheduler! She needed a little pep talk!

Once the doctor realized that I would not budge until I got the US done, she went and pulled some strings and got the test ordered. "What was so hard about that?" This was after all, a huge hospital. There were plenty of ways to get an ultrasound completed. If she did not order it, I planned to go into the regular ED (Emergency Department) and pull some strings of my own. To think, this woman actually looked at me nonchalantly and said, "You still have time to start the medication according to studies." She did so with a 'don't worry about it' look on her face as she attempted to shrug the whole thing off. "Forget you and your studies! That's not what we discussed!" "Unless you people are dumb and blind, this test needed to be ordered right now!" I waited around the area for a couple of hours until it was time to get the ultrasound completed. It really wasn't that doctor's fault, it was the whole team, especially that lazy scheduler, whom I believe did not pass the information along. She could have told the team about it if she had difficulties making the appointment. Instead, she chose to just sit on it; as if this wasn't an important task. I cannot stand being treated that way.

My initial appointment was at nine thirty in the mornings. I waited around till five in the evening to have that ultrasound. Basically, I spent an entire day just for one thing. I did not pout though. I let it all roll off my back. "At least it was being done", I comforted myself. I'll get a better group of doctors next time. Hopefully, somebody can fully please me at some point. The moment came for the ultrasound to be completed and the pictures that resulted were amazing! At eight weeks, you could see the fetus looking like a tiny tadpole. We managed to actually see tiny webbed hands and feet. The webbed hands waved at me. I even got a chance to see the yolk sac. Unbelievable! So early on, so much could be observed. More importantly, the fetus was properly placed within the uterus. That meant that I could begin taking the subcutaneous anticoagulant Lovenox.

To my surprise, the doctor called me that same night to confirm the results and place the order for the Lovenox. "Now she was moving fast!" That was one hurdle out of the way and many more to come. "Why did I have to go through all of that?" "I simply could not understand why these people did that?" It hurt me to this day, thinking about it. Now, all I had to do was pick up my medication and start my new daily routine.

TWENTY-FOUR
REAL THIS TIME

As the current pregnancy advanced, I became extremely nauseous. I would vomit regularly and not only in the morning either. I would be almost done eating at the table and suddenly feel lumps of food regurgitating upwards my esophagus. At that moment, I tried sitting upright to assist with reverting the direction of the movement. Often, I would be praying for the meal to stay down. Nevertheless, it came up anyways. By the time the gush of puke exited my mouth, I had no choice but to throw everything back up in the plate in front of me. I really did not have a chance to run to a more appropriate place. The only good thing was that we used paper plates. Our ceramic plates were used mostly when guests visited to save on water bill and the bothersome dish washing. This nausea was so regular and frequent that I feared eating. I tried to eat a little bit at a time so not to induce the vomiting. I would drink only a little bit of water after eating and continued the method of sitting erect for at least half an hour to stop my food from regurgitating. I tried to give it a chance to digest.

One other episode involved me laying down in bed. I had recently finished eating and felt extremely fatigued. "Now, I was aware that I needed to either sit upright post eating or walk around a bit to expedite the digesting process but, felt so sleepy that I couldn't." Despite the fact that I sat in the kitchen for a little bit prior to laying down in bed, the puking episode got me anyways. I found myself ready to barf as I was rotated from one side to another. I tried to speed walk to the bathroom to alleviate myself but, was unsuccessful. A gush of disgusting food particles mixed with bile flew out of my mouth and unto to floor of my bedroom! Yuck! How sickening! There was no stopping this repulsive phenomenon.

Afterward, I had to clean the entire thing up. "Fun times!" "More work for the pregnant, tired and irritable woman."

At some point, my husband and I decided that it would be best if I took my medication a half hour to an hour before consuming any food. That way, I would retain the medication and not throw it up. As it turned out, I was able to taste the pills that I took when I vomited. This signified that the meds were not being consumed or digested. Knowing that the medications may not be getting absorbed worried us tremendously. It was impertinent that I received the benefits of all of my meds but, especially my baby Aspirin. This medication was crucial to not only the survival of the fetus but, to mines as well.

Another equally disgusting symptom involved spitting mucus out of my mouth all day. It was as if I was overfilled with phlegm and had to constantly empty out my body. I found myself needing to carry an empty water bottle wherever I went just for hawking. Since I was at home most of the time, my room became filled with bottles of mucus. The containers were filled at different levels. If I used one bottle and didn't have to spit for a while, the container may have become contaminated. There was no reason to reopen it and experience that horrible, spoiled, rotten smell. This occurred especially when the bottles were left in my car. The hot, blazing sun caused the saliva to spoil even faster. Often, the bottles were a one-time use.

The constant spitting was absolutely sickening to me. I remembered hearing stories of Haitian women experiencing that symptom of pregnancy. My mother always said that she never actually had that happen to her. It was kind of looked down upon; particularly those women who just spit in the street. It was classier to do as I was doing and having a container to privately use whenever the urge would come. I myself, had moments where I didn't have any clean, empty bottles with me while driving. I tried spitting out the car window, only to have sputum splash back in my face. Then there were moments where I missed the ground altogether and mucus would land on the side steps of my vehicle. I didn't like that much. I knew that I would have to step over it when getting out of the car.

Despite being severely annoyed by all of these happenings, I was thankful. Yes! Believe it or not, I felt thankful to be throwing up wherever I would go. I felt grateful to be spitting in every empty water bottle that I could find. These occurrences were very satisfying. The fact that they were happening assured me that I was having a normal pregnancy. They indicated that my hormone levels were correct and working accordingly.

The thing was, during my first pregnancy, I never had any of these symptoms. I felt nauseous and had some food aversion but, never anything as significant as what I was experiencing now. Indeed, it might seem odd to others for me to think like this but, that is how I felt. At least now, I had actual, visual evidence of a pregnancy.

TWENTY-FIVE
SWEET FAMILY CARE

With everything now looking up, other members of our close family started suspecting that we were expecting. They noticed the changes, the new upbeat attitudes and not to mention the rapid weight gain. They instantly detected the great news! They seemed more excited than us at times. My mother and father were both ready to be grandparents and this was their opportunity.

My mother began to smother me with all types of gifts. She came over one night and handed to me numerous gowns that she specially ordered for me. There were many different colors; one for each day it appeared. I had a red gown, one yellow, a green colored one with beautiful, detailed embroidery and one pink gown that had a nice, thick, warm sweater to match. They were very lovely! Each gown had a great length to it and could be worn outside close to the house.

In addition to those colorful gowns, she purchased some rare, strong quality shoes. She only brought from a pricey catalog that delivered long lasting products. She really was a woman of great and expansive taste. The shoes were fabulous! She gifted me a golden slipper with tassels and a white leather shoe, which matched a cute white lace dress that I previously own. I also received a comfortable black pair of leather shoes. They were the type that people with feet problems often bought. They looked the safest out of the three. Although, with the hot summer heat approaching, I didn't see myself wearing them much. They would certainly have good usage later though. Plus, I knew that there would be more.

My father was also very excited to hear this wonderful news. He had been waiting impatiently to hear me say that I was with child. Upon knowing, he jokingly asked my husband on a regular basis, "If he was making sure the baby was well fed." He would visually assess my stomach for adequate growth, noting that my progress was quite different from my previous pregnancy of 24 weeks. It was better, much, much better actually. As a big man himself, he strongly encouraged eating as much as possible to promote a good weight gain for the baby. It was understandable why that concerned him in particular. The prior incident involved inadequate fetal growth. My father did not want to have that repeated. I prayed not to see that ever again either.

TWENTY-SIX

NO WORK

In the meantime, I still had not returned to work. I continued to be on my leave. Unfortunately for me, it was unpaid. Those bastards would not give me any money for my time off. Maybe it was because I hadn't been at the job but for a little over a year. I still had bills to pay though. I needed something to subsidize my income or my husband's. I tried to file for short term disability, which: "I forgot that I had been paying for." The form was sent to me and I told my doctor about it, since she needed to sign it. At another physician's visit with one of the doctors, I reminded her that I needed her to sign the short-term disability forms and her response was stunning. She flat out refused. She swatted her hand as if to say, "I'm not doing that." She explained that "She didn't want to risk her license." The swatting though, was what really made me mad. "Did she have to be so rude?" "Did she have any kind of home training."

Later during that same visit, my husband asked her about nutritional intake for a pregnant woman. He wanted to know what I should and should not be eating. He was acting as a concerned husband. In response, this doctor goes off with the hand swatting again. "What in the world was this?" "What was up with the rude hand gesture! You shouldn't be talking to a dog like that!" I wanted to take her hand and swat her face with it. I never realized that this young woman was like that. I do recall her coming in briefly during my stillbirth, swatting away. I thought that it was due to the stress of deciding rather or not to have surgery on my small uterus. It would be risky and cause me to bleed tremendously. Plus, I had only been with the practice for a short time back then. It never really occurred to me that this young lady had a bad attitude. When I first spoke to her during this current pregnancy, she did appear to be under a lot of pressure. I wondered if she had been getting a lot of complaints from other clients. She appeared that much tense. Plus, I never realized how much she spoke like a school girl. It was "Like oh my God, I can't do that." "Oh my God" this, "Oh my God" that. What had I gotten myself into?

Truth be told, I only liked one physician that I met out of that practice. This one woman was an experienced mother. She was the person who delivered my son whom was stillbirth. She was very patient and caring. She was also very confident in what she was doing. It appeared that she was a senior in the practice because the rude, young lady at one point, acted scared to override one of her orders. This doctor that delivered my son also took the time to talk with me briefly about plans for another pregnancy. Unlike the others, she seemed to really care. It's something that was not apparent with the rest of the staff members.

Just like that, with one hand swatting I would not be getting paid to stay home. "I wondered if the first male doctor at the other practice would have helped me out?" He most likely would have. This man had more experience than this young, rude, female and wasn't as stiff. He may have been a little more understanding in this situation. After all, I was high risk with prior losses and I had a job that put me at greater risk for injury. There were plenty of reasons for me to stay home. Plus, I was at the time truly injured secondary to my employment. Looks like I'll have to find another way around this mess. I'm sure I'll think of something.

TWENTY-SEVEN

AT HOME

Hanging out at home and keeping up with work related stuff, kept me busy. I spent my days going back and forth with the job making sure that I was still allotted my health insurance. I was after all on a leave. I had not resigned my position. In the meantime, I hoped to find another position. I was advised not to get a new job by my parents and to just concentrate on the pregnancy at hand. My father repeatedly reminded me that I was advanced in age now and was at a disadvantage. He wanted to remind me that now that I was in my thirties, I had a less chance of successfully having a child. Therefore, if I was pregnant, then I should take full advantage of that. He didn't care if I gave birth to this child with just a piece of bread to my name. His only goal was to make sure that I stayed put at home and grow this baby. Work would be available later.

As hard as it was for me to stay home and not work or have any sort of activities, I decided that I would make a sacrifice and do it. I certainly did not want to go and risk this pregnancy. Plus, I had to remember that I was not like everyone else. My body was a bit more fragile than that of other women. It was important that I took extra precautions.

For my husband though, it was a little more difficult. He seemed unaccustomed to the stress of handling all the affairs in the home. He appeared ever so worried about everything that had to do with money. He tried not to become anxious whenever he had to spend money for anything. At some point, I wouldn't do food shopping with him. I would go with him and let him buy whatever he thought that we needed. Later, I would go shopping for any extra items that I wanted during the week. There was no need to have any miscommunication during our little shopping trips. I knew he was adopting to new responsibilities and I wanted to stay out of the way of that extreme stress. Now, I understood why some women say that they would never stop working and let the man handle everything. Him and I were on two different pages when it came to money. I wasn't afraid to spend it when I had to, as long as it was for something important. For him, he wanted to hold on tight to it for some kind of perceived emergency that may never happen. My model was that another job was always around the corner. Fortunately, with my nursing career, that fact was true. I never had a difficult time getting a job. I had a bachelor's degree, and did not have much to worry about. I experienced life much differently than he did.

In reality, I was a very frugal woman who occasionally splurged. My own mother often became mad at me for that very reason. To her, I was one of the cheapest persons that she knew. At the same time though, she was the kind of person that wouldn't be satisfied until you spent your last dime. Even though I had some money, it was the result of extremely hard-work. Knowing that I didn't plan on doing the same job forever, I was careful not to spend recklessly. I knew that one day I would stop working for one reason or another.

TWENTY-EIGHT

GENDER

Since the pregnancy was progressing normally, we were able as a couple to focus on more fun things. Wondering what would be the sex of the baby was now common talk in our home. My husband wanted a boy. He said that he would feel more comfortable with his own sex. I agreed with him that a boy would be wonderful since, they love their mothers so much. I loved how boys always protected their mothers even as a little toddler. I wanted my husband to be happy since he seemed to really want a child. Undoubtedly, I wanted a child as well but, I did not believe in my heart that this child was a boy. We already had our opportunity at bringing a baby boy into this world. God was now switching up the options.

For starter, I had this intuitive feeling that this baby was a female. Plus, all of the symptoms from the current pregnancy were very different from my prior pregnancy when I was carrying a boy. The excess of nausea and vomiting led me to think that I was producing way more hormones than before. I suspected that I was producing female hormones. I heard once that when a woman carries a female fetus, they tend to produce more hormones like estrogen and progesterone. The woman would produce both for herself and the female embryo.

Either way, it really didn't matter to me what the sex of the baby was. As long as the child was healthy, I would be content with whatever God gave me. Having been in some very disappointing situations before, all that I wanted was happiness. I would accept it in whatever shape or form that God brought it to me. I tried to convince my husband that a little girl would love her daddy immensely. Little girls also protected their fathers. They protected them as a toddler from their mothers. Either way, we would soon find out. We would know exactly what we were having in a few, short weeks.

TWENTY-NINE
PREGNANCY PAIN

Waking up from bed one day towards the end of my third month, I realized that I was having difficulties walking. I had never felt that pain before. I had no clue as to why or where this pain was coming from. The only thing that was apparent was that I had to take little steps to get around. I was literally sliding from one step to another. I did some research and found out what was causing the aching. It was round ligament pain. This was a term I could now add to my new vocabulary list. I understood the method and reasoning behind the pain and it made total sense to me.

I would complain to my mother about it and she looked at me like "Duh." "Pregnancy hurts", she said "You're going to feel pain." "How was I supposed to know?" I had never experienced a real pregnancy before and definitely never had any normal symptoms prior either. The only things that I knew about we're losses. She, being the experienced one in this field, told me exactly what I needed to do. She suggested that I elevated my legs when I was sleeping to alleviate the pain. That way, the muscle would not be stretched to a maximum all the time. I tried the method that she recommended and it actually worked. I felt less pain and had a better time walking around after that.

Finally, I called my doctor to tell her what was going on and she clarified that I would benefit from wearing a belt to help support the expanding uterus. I purchased one of those but, couldn't figure out how to properly apply it. The company that I got it from sent it through a third party. It looked like something that was already used. There was not even tag, box or anything. Therefore, I couldn't use the product nor return it. Thank goodness though, the pain subsided slowly on its own. I figured, once the round ligaments became accustomed to the growth of the uterus, the pain would decrease.

Oddly enough, I missed the pain once it was gone. Once again, it made me feel happy to be experiencing these symptoms. I felt great joy to have pain and discomfort like other pregnant women. It was very comforting for me. It reassured me that growth was taking place. Unlike my very first pregnancy, where I felt no such discomfort. I was now going through real pregnancy experiences and real pregnancy symptoms. Now, I could honestly say that "I felt like a real pregnant woman!"

THIRTY
NAMING

Now that everything seemed in order, we decided that it was time to find a meaningful and creative name for our child. We wanted the name not to only be cute and easily pronounced but, meaningful. We especially wanted our baby's name to be from good examples found in the Bible. Our child should be blessed before she even entered this world. Better yet, since I had such a difficult time bearing children, I too needed all of the blessings that I could get. I asked the elders in the congregation to pray for me and to have the entire congregation pray on my behalf, my baby and my husband. I truly felt that they had done and we're still doing exactly that. I felt blessed to be at the stage that I was in. My husband and I became so excited everytime we heard the baby's new weight. We both had never been through such a wonderful experience. We never felt this much positivity in our lives. We only wished that it would continue. Our hope was that we experienced positivity and happiness until the arrival of this blessed child.

During our weekly family Bible study, we prayed on finding the best possible name. Of course, we wanted it to start with the letter

"E." It was a tradition in my family that all children be named after the first letter of the father's name. We thought of a few different options. Esther was at the top of my list. I always said that if I had a girl, I would name her Esther. I remember reading the book of Esther while in high school and falling in love with her. "What a strong, beautiful and courageous woman!" Esther managed to save an entire group of people by her swift, bold and quick thinking. I admired her greatly and wanted my daughter to have the same characteristics. I wanted her to grow knowing that her name had significance and wasn't some made up collage with no meaning. Her name would inspire her to be the best person that she possibly could be. Despite loving the name Esther and all that it stood for, we decided to keep our options open.

"How many names were there to choose from that started with the letter E?" There was Ezekiel, Ezra, Esther, Ecclesiastes, Eli, Enoch, Ebenezer, Elizabeth and quite a few more. None of these seemed to catch our attention though. We were looking for something to satisfy the both of us equally.

At last, my husband ran into a really good one, "Emmanuel." Now I know what you're thinking: "That name doesn't began with an 'E', it starts with the letter 'I'!" Even though that might be true in

English, in other languages like French, that name was spelled differently. "Emmanuel" did begin with an 'E'.

That beautiful name sounded common and kind of unexciting at first. As a matter of fact, I could remember on numerous occasions promising myself not to ever name my child by that exact name for different reasons. Neither the male or the female version suited me. That was until we researched the meaning of this simple name. As it turned out, Emmanuel was not a name at all but, a title. It wasn't just any label though but, one of great significance. Emmanuel was a title that relates to Jesus Christ. It meant God is with us. What a blessing!

The name was perfect in every sense. This was it, we would name her Emmanuella! Our child would have a great start to life. We, as parents, would do our best to reinforce the meaning of that name. We were so thrilled to have found this wonderful name! We could now concentrate on all good things to come!

THIRTY-ONE
FUTURE

Focusing on the future felt so good. I was waiting impatiently for the arrival of my beautiful baby girl. I continued receiving care at the private doctor with my private health insurance. My job was still providing me health insurance at my expense. I was thankful though, to have their insurance with the heavy copay. It certainly was better than nothing.

At close to six months pregnant, I made the decision to switch to a new health insurance program. I wanted to transition into government health insurance which paid for everything without copay. Since I was on an unpaid leave, I could no longer afford the heavy charges. With the government insurance, I wouldn't need to worry about making any additional spending. Plus, I would still be seen at the same hospital. I would deliver at the same previously planned facility. Not much would change. The only thing was that I would see a different group of doctors. The current group was not all of that anyways, with the exception of one. Most of the doctors there didn't seem to understand holistic care. They only treated the cause at hand, not the patient as a whole.

Around the time of the transitioning process, my anxiety got the best of me. Despite deciding not to work at all, I tried looking for an easier, less difficult new job and was hired. I was about 22 weeks along and wore a big blazer jacket with a big purse. I kept the purse on my lap during the entire interview. No one was suspicious except for one person when I was leaving the office. She looked confused as if she couldn't make out if I was just fat or what? Everything would have worked out if it was not for the pre-employment physical. The nurse practitioner there was ridiculously thorough. It seemed that she may have picked up that I was pregnant and it caused me to worry. I thought that she would not pass me on the assessment. Surprisingly, she approved me and sent me on my way; leaving me still uncertain if she knew or not.

Later, at a different date, I received a phone call from the company regarding my MMR (Measles, Mumps and Rubella) titer being too low. The lady on the phone told me that I needed another dose of vaccination to replenish it. This company was obviously a really good company if it went through all of that trouble for pre-employment screening. I hadn't had an in-depth examination like this one since I first started nursing. Evidently, I was unable to receive that type of vaccination during pregnancy. I immediately declined and made the human resource department aware of my inability to work. I was completely honest with them and they were very understanding. They told me to just reapply once I was ready to work.

The same day of the pre-employment physical, I went to my doctor's office to have a routine examination. Even though I knew everything was fine with the baby, I felt worried as always. "Thank goodness the doctor that I saw that day was the one doctor that I enjoyed seeing." She always had a very calm and relaxed demeanor. I wondered if today she could do a quick ultrasound like they sometimes do. I desperately wanted to see my baby.

Once I was seen, my favorite doctor examined me and said that the baby was perfect. She only listened to the heart beat and assessed my fundal height. She told me that everything was going fine with the baby. The fact that she was most concerned about was how anxious I appeared. She questioned if I was scared? I answered her with tears in my eyes. "Of course! I was terrified!" With three pregnancy losses under my belt, I was mortified! The doubts were inevitable. "Would I actually have this child? Would I carry this child full term? Would I suffer that horrific preeclampsia again?" She was very sweet but, stern towards me. She reassured me once more that: "The baby was perfect and that I had nothing to worry about." Her uplifting words made me feel better for the moment.

After that attempt of working again, I made the firm decision to sit my butt down and just focus on my baby. A job would be there for me when I was done giving birth. It would be there even way afterward. I needed to just relax and not worry about money. At some points in one's life you have to take it easy. Pregnancy was one of those moments. Bringing a human into this world required making sacrifices and it would all be worth it at the end.

THIRTY-TWO
NEW INSURANCE

Oh boy! It was transitioning time! I was now trying to change from private health insurance to medical assistance. This process should be smooth. Now at 23 weeks pregnant, I hadn't had an income for six months. I had already spoken to the counselor at the hospital about what steps I needed to take months prior. We went over what paperwork I would need to bring in and at what moment. I felt ready to go through the process. I was all prepared for the switch, so I thought.

It didn't bother me to be on public assistance for a little bit. Some people judge and see it as laziness but, it is a program that's in place for a reason. If I don't stop working, I'm likely to lose another child just like the others. It was important that I paced myself and made sure I did everything right this time around. Therefore, using what programs the government had in place seemed like a great option for me. If you think about it, people on medical assistance seem to be doing the right way. A lot of these women use the public benefit available, have many children and then go to school. Usually, when they attend school, they use whatever funding the government has to offer. They spend no money of their own. Later, they end up being the same women working as Registered Nurses and even Nurse Practitioners. They know exactly what they are doing. Plus, those co-payments were killing me who had no money. In addition, I would be delivering at the very same facility either ways so, who cared.

When I at last went to get the switch completed, the young lady who assisted with obtaining health insurance was either nervous, conceded, rude or uneducated in her field. The fact that my husband didn't have all of his paperwork, she advised me that I might not be able to receive the medical assistance that I needed. I thought that she sounded very silly. "Of course, I would be able to get the full benefits." "There were people who came here from other countries without their husbands and still received care", I reminded her. She told me snobbishly, that my husband was here, so it wasn't the same case for me. I wanted her to keep her mouth shut. "Just be quiet", I thought. I ignored what she said and took all my paperwork and went to a public clinic. Back again to my favorite spot.

Once at the public facility, I spoke to a counselor and she helped me out tremendously. She seemed a bit hesitant about my husband's documents not been available too but, did not push me away like the prior girl. She filed the form, took all the information that I had and told me that she would contact me once the application was approved or if she needed any further information.

In the meantime, I ended up making an appointment at another local hospital in case something did not pan out. That hospital did not have a problem seeing me without any health insurance. It was more of a community hospital. In reality, it was my old stomping ground. I used to work there when I had my first miscarriage. They were good for helping people out with low income that were underinsured or uninsured. Once I was seen there, they took good care of me. They drew labs, assessed my vitals and ordered me one month's supply of the Lovenox that I so desperately needed. They did so at a very, very discounted price through their own pharmacy. I was extremely thankful for their help. Unlike the other private hospital, they did not leave me out in the streets. They did not tell me that I couldn't make an appointment or be seen without health insurance. This hospital truly proved to be available for those in the community when they were in need.

Two to three weeks later, I received that phone call from my counselor at the clinic confirming my acceptance. My card came in the mail only a few days later. "Just like I thought." "Why wouldn't the government give me the health benefit that I needed?" "All of the taxes I paid over the years!?" Back to the private hospital I went where my care was first initiated.

THIRTY-THREE
PRIVATE HOSPITAL

Happy to be where I needed to be, I obtained an appointment for the next week. Through questioning by the nurse, I explained how I was pushed away and out in the streets by staff of the hospital. Honestly, I felt terrible about all of the behaviors. I did not want to be spiteful but, wanted to make changes for others. I was a very high-risk patient. I should have never been made to feel as if I would not be able to receive care; especially, in this grand country we live in. No one should ever feel like that.

Once everything was back on track, I felt relieved. I was now receiving the care that I needed and more. I now had a nurse coordinator to guide my entire care. There was a social worker that assisted me with everything that I needed, even those unrelated to health issues. Basically, if I needed a car seat, she would make sure I got it. If I needed clothes, food, or even a crib, she promised to find a way for me to get me those items. Of course, I took full advantage of all of the offers. I even asked the social worker to write down a list of all the community resources available. I wanted information on all programs that were giving out free stuff for mother's and babies. "Why not enjoy this while it lasted?" "Take advantage of all that was offered, while I was at it." "Once I went back to work, all of this was over!" The only thing that I had to worry about now was bringing home my brand-new baby girl. I'm so glad that this current office focused on holistic care. Unlike my prior private practice doctors, these individuals knew what I needed. This was exactly what I was looking for!

THIRTY-FOUR
PANICKING

At some point I started to panic. "What was I going to do with this child?" "What was I going to teach her?" I knew that I wanted her to know God and to live as a true Christian, but I started having doubt in myself. I wondered if I was educated enough in God's word to guide my child successfully. As these thoughts came into my mind, I decided that now was the time to start reading the good Holy Book from top to bottom. I mean, I was already in the habit of reading along weekly but, I wanted to focus more. I started from the very beginning, the book of Genesis. I continued reading and found great comfort in doing so. I already knew the stories but, wanted to revise everything that I was taught throughout my entire life. I read the entire story of Moses leading the Israelites towards the land that Jehovah had promised his people. I revised in depth the story of Abraham and his wife Sarah and how Jehovah used them in his service. Sarah served as an obedient and respectful wife to Abraham, always allowing him to take the lead. I didn't just read to know the information thought, I meditated on their applications too.

I imagined that if my daughter had a problem of some kind, I would use examples found in the Bible to help her. For instance, the story of Joseph was a prime example of forgiveness. Despite being sold into slavery by his own brothers, Joseph did not hold a grudge against them. He did not show resentment when he later saw them coming to buy food during the great famine in Egypt. Joseph acknowledged that Jehovah sent him ahead of the others to preserve life. He readily provided all of them, including his father Jacob with food and housing needed for them to survive. Other wonderful examples included Noah, who was a great servant of God. Despite being bullied, belittled and mocked by those around him at the time, Noah graciously listened to what Jehovah commanded him. Noah and his family were the only ones to preach the coming of the great flood. They tried to save as many lives as possible. He was not embarrassed nor afraid to do such a work. Noah and his family had a great relationship with Jehovah God and they did not allow anyone to discourage them from doing what they knew was right. This was so even if it meant looking like outcasts.

Knowing all of these examples, would prove to be beneficial when raising my precious baby. Plus, I did not want her to think that I did not know what I was talking about. With prayer, guidance, the help of my husband and other friends, I hoped that I would be able to raise my child in the right lane of life.

THIRTY-FIVE
HOME

At home, we were trying to get things ready and in order. There was an extra room for the baby but, it was not exactly a "baby's room" quite yet. A lot of changes and alterations had to be made. For starter, a piece of the ceiling had begun leaking again. Ironically, only the ceiling in that room leaked. While sleeping in bed there one night, I felt something wet. When I woke up, I noticed it was more of a puddle. I thought: "Could it be amniotic fluid?" I was skeptical but, realized that the puddle was not underneath me or barely really touching me unless I switched positions. It was impossible to be amniotic fluid. I concluded that it was the roof leaking again after three years post repair. For some reason or another, I ignored that first leak. I'm not sure if it was fatigue, despair, round ligament pains or frustration but, I hoped that it would just go away.

Eventually though, it rained heavy again during the month of May and caused the leaking to recommence. This time, I managed to get up, get a bucket and placed it under where the now heavy outflow was happening. It was impossible to ignore this flowing river.

Right away we called the roofing company that repaired the original problem three years prior. I still had the original documents and proof of a 25-year warranty. Although, I'm sure that there would be a loop hole for them to jump out of. I made the call and asked them to come and fix the thing right away. No doubt I got the run around and had to call again. By the time they got to looking at the damage it was already June. Then all they agreed to do was coat it for a price. I wasn't convinced if that would really fix the problem. We waited out for a while, mostly because we didn't want to spend the money that we didn't have. Plus, I wanted a permanent fix.

At last, through a good, honest and dependable friend, I got the name and number of a good roofer. This particular friend, I knew to be detailed and pesky when it came to evaluating people and their work performances. I knew he wouldn't mislead me. Like an angel descending from heaven, the young contractor had the same ideas that I had. Instead of coating, why not replace the damaged portion of the roof and formed it so that the water no longer pooled in that spot. That way, water would no longer leak through the roof but divert off of the roof. He even offered to fix the damaged ceiling. The entire thing would cost the same amount offered to me to have the roof coated. Once that was done, we could move forward with renovation of the room for the newborn. In due time, there would be no more raining of any sort in that room.

THIRTY-SIX
LOOKING BACK

It was amazing how far I had come. From losing my first child at 24 weeks to having difficulty conceiving and now in my third trimester awaiting the arrival of my beautiful daughter. Undoubtedly, I had some uncertainties. There was always something in the back of my mind that made me question the reality of this outcome. "Would I actually go full term?" "Would I have early onset preeclampsia like before?" "Should I bring my hopes up or should I remain neutral so that I am not disappointed if the unthinkable happens?" I recalled telling a friend about two to three months into the pregnancy that I didn't feel excited. She had to convince me to get excited. No matter what, at least I was trying again and giving way to new hope.

It was important that I used all that had happened as a strength and not as a weakness. I should not think of my failures in the past as a cause to doubt the positives that were happening to me in the present. My husband helped me to think straight too. He continued to support this new era in our lives by always reminding me of how far we had come. He would always say, "Be thankful to Jehovah for where we are." "Don't focus on the past but, on the now." It was satisfying to know that I was not doing this alone. I was not taking this journey by myself but, with someone that equally wanted to achieve great results. My husband and I both wanted to successfully bring our child into this world. I was blessed to have someone that helped keep me positive.

THIRTY-SEVEN

DOUBTS

The doubts that I had, eventually led me to have multiple L and D visits. One such visit occurred when I noticed fluid leaking down my legs from my vagina after a shower. Usually, I used an old shower chair of my grandmother to sit while I washed. This one day, it just so happened that once I stood up, fluid started leaking down my legs. It wasn't fluid from the shower because I had already wiped myself considerably prior. Instinctively, I thought of the worse. I thought that is was amniotic fluid. At a second glance, I thought that maybe it was the menstrual period affect. Similar to when a menstruating woman sits down for too long, once she stood up abruptly, her period would leak even more. Also, I felt like it was my bladder emptying in small spurts. Confident, that it was nothing, I let the situation go for about a day or two. Then for one reason or another, I began to worry if I should have called the doctor to be safe. Feeling anxious, I made the phone call and through her suggestion, admitted myself to L and D. I'm sure those women were happy to see me. The doctor took a good look at my cervix and determined that everything was fine. No openings were found, no leaking noted either. She did inform me though, that if that happened again, I was to come in as quickly as possible. She explained to me that a leaking cervix was a life and death situation for both myself and the baby.

Another time, I went to labor and delivery when I found out that my liver enzymes were slightly elevated. The results came to me from the other local, community hospital that I temporarily switched to. I felt worried and took actions into my own hands. I knew the seriousness of these results. In addition, I had a throbbing headache and wanted to be sure the two weren't related. I checked my blood pressure and heart rate at home but, decided to rely on the symptoms. I was anxious so, I concluded that the anxiety might be the reason why my blood pressure was elevated and that it wasn't a real reading. I rushed to the L and D and had myself reassessed. The same lab works were repeated and my vital signs obtained. This was the moment where certain individuals seemed irritable. They acted as if I was making things up. I did not pay them any attention. I knew my medical background better than anybody else. I knew what to take seriously and what to take lightly. This case was not to be taken nonchalantly at all. Despite having explained to the nurse how no one believed me with my first major blood clot and how I almost died, she still responded annoyingly when my blood pressure was in the 100's over 80's. She even sucked her teeth. "Better to be sure then to be sorry", I said. Sadly, due to my skepticism and neediness to have this pregnancy be successful, there would be more trips to come.

A few weeks later, as I entered my third trimester, I made sure that I did my kick counts daily. I would assure that there were ten or more movements or kicks during a two-hour period each day. I would lay on my left side and patiently count each movement. One of those days, I didn't recall feeling movements as I did before. My issue was that as I became 29 weeks along, I felt a couple of huge kicks that were visibly noticeable. Later, during that same week, I did not observe the same strength of kicks. I waited until the next day and still nothing of the same caliber. I notified the on-call doctor and he told me that if I wanted to, then I could come to be seen. The option was presented to me so I took him up on it.

Upon arriving on the floor, I knew some people recognized me. One of them was a wonderful nurse that I actually enjoyed seeing. I was thrilled that she was working that day. I did the routine and gave my urine sample and changed into a gown. I laid on the bed and waited for someone to come and hook me up to the machines. Once all of that was done, we decided that the baby was moving more than adequate and that everything was going smoothly. The nurse practitioner that was on board actually did a quick ultrasound to prove to me that the baby was fine. My little darling was chilling in there. She looked like someone that was resting in bed for the day. I was told later that at that stage, the baby mostly relaxed and tasted everything that mamma ate. She looked like that was exactly what she was doing too. With her thumb in her mouth and her lips smacking, she was definitely tasting some delicious, sweet, red apples. This little girl must be sick of me constantly putting her through tests and assessments. All that she wanted to do was kick back and relax.

THIRTY-EIGHT
HOME AGAIN

Deciding to finally take it easy and start thinking positively, I commenced looking at décor options for the nursery. I went to my favorite paint shop and began looking at paint color selections. I was thinking of pink walls. I didn't want bright pink or even obvious pink but, something subtle. The room needed something that was inviting and not offensive. If I had to be in a bright, pink room for even a short period of time, I would find it very nauseating. It really would not be an enjoyable experience. Having thought of that, I wanted the room to be enjoyable for my child, myself and anyone who entered it. I decided on a wall color that was a cute mixture of cream and some pink. That way, it would match the wall colors of the rest of the house.

In addition, I took a peek at some wallpaper choices too. I considered this before but without really seeing any up close. I saw some different style wallpapers online and loved how unique and intricate they appeared once installed. Although, I had not considered the amount of work it took to install these beautiful masterpieces. My husband would have to glue the wallpaper, if I chose the type that was already in colored design. If I chose the ones that were elevated prints, he would have to glue the paper to the wall and paint over them to add color. After realizing that, I decided to opt out of wallpaper altogether. It was too much work. My husband was working very hard and I didn't want to add more strain to his already busy routine. The baby could decide on what she wanted when she got older. For now, I just wanted to please the eyes of the adults and not burden the eyes of the child.

THIRTY-NINE

CURRENT

Now with a healthy growing baby in my belly, I was only awaiting and counting the days. I was thankful to Jehovah God for having made it this far. I could feel my baby kick on a daily basis. She even reacted to noises that she heard from the environment. Now that I was not working, I basically rested most of the days. Most days, I felt so exhausted that I had to crawl to the bed to 'pass out.' Some days, the temperature got so high that I wondered: "How on earth would I have been able to drive around to people's houses and assess them as a home care RN (Registered Nurse)?" Not to mention, the neighborhood that I was going to be assigned to was not the safest. Upon hearing the name Kensington, I sighed but decided to give it a go. I would have deeply regretted taking that position.

Kensington was a filthy, drug addict's paradise. It's an area that I rarely went to unless I had to drive through to get to another location. Usually, when I did drive through, I would stare in dismay. It was pretty disbelieving the type of people that you mostly saw there. The living arrangements and lifestyles were dangerous to say the least.

One day, my husband drove me by an area that I never knew existed. He always spoke of it before but, I honestly could never imagine. It was astonishing to see long rows of people living under a bridge in tents. Literally, this was happening in my own city. I guess I was taking the scenic route all of those years. He continued driving to another location to show me more. As we approached, all I saw was a sea of people that you just knew were high on some kind of drug. These people were living in the streets! The drug epidemic was really strong in the city of Philadelphia. I didn't need anyone to tell me that, I could see it with my own two eyes. "Can you imagine me doing home care in an area like that?" It was obvious why they hired me and offered to pay me a bucket load of money. Who would want to deal with these unsafe conditions!

FORTY

SAFE AT HOME

Safe at home and advancing normally, I continued to be thankful. We were only weeks away from seeing a marvel! Each week that would arise, my husband and I would look up information on what details were happening with the baby and mommy. Even though the present week was not completely over, we would start looking up the upcoming week. The excitement highly got to us!

We were deeply praying that the weeks would fly by and out pop out our gorgeous little mamma with full lips and all. I just knew she would be the most stunning being ever. I knew I was, and she looked exactly like me. Her beauty was clearly visible on the ultrasound. I hoped that she had a mixture of both mines and her father's personality. We wanted her to be outgoing and talkative like her father with a shy, sweet balance like her mother. I couldn't imagine a child with a closed-in personality. Plans were already in place to help her overcome that obstacle if she needed it. My baby would be comfortable in her skin. She would manage to get along with everyone and respect others for who they were. Confidence was what I wanted for her and confidence was what I believed she would inherent.

Now 31 weeks pregnant on the 31st of July, I was steadily counting down the moment till I gave birth! Yes! Birth! I can honestly say that this time around. I can finally look forward to having my baby squeeze right out of me. She would scream and cry until I held her. This child would come with an open mouth to grab my nipples and suck on them. I smiled at the thought. Actually, I laughed with great joy to myself. "This was going to be a reality for me!" This moment was something that both my husband and I couldn't wait to see with our own eyes.

We had done everything that we were supposed to. We made the ultimate sacrifices. I stopped working and stayed home. My husband took over the household, fear and all. He managed to take care of business despite feeling terrified and incompetent. He proved to himself that he could indeed do what he did not believe in himself to be capable of doing. This is what our story was all about. We Believed in ourselves and knew that we could achieve the unthinkable. We were waiting to prove to ourselves and everyone around us that we can achieve success!

www.ingramcontent.com/pod-product-compliance
Lightning Source LLC
Chambersburg PA
CBHW020644220526
45464CB00001B/291